CHINESE RED YEAST RICE

A Remarkable Compound for the Promotion of Healthy Cholesterol Levels

RITA ELKINS, M.H.

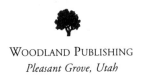

WOODLAND PUBLISHING
Pleasant Grove, Utah

The information in this book is for educational purposes only and is not recommended as a means of diagnosing or treating an illness. All matters concerning physical and mental health should be supervised by a health practitioner knowledgeable in treating that particular condition. Neither the publisher nor author directly or indirectly dispense medical advice, nor do they prescribe any remedies or assume any responsibility for those who choose to treat themselves.

Table of Contents

Introduction

Over the last few years, several natural substances capable of lowering potentially harmful blood fats and cholesterol levels have emerged. While no one is suggesting that we can promote healthy cholesterol levels by taking a "magic pill," nature has provided us with specific compounds capable of augmenting dietary and lifestyle changes for improved cardiovascular health. Unquestionably, one of the most impressive of these is a compound extracted from red yeast rice, a fermented food substance which has been traditionally used for its red-coloring capabilities in meats and other foods. In addition to its pigment value, red yeast rice offers some very valuable therapeutic benefits. In fact, it is the source of certain compounds, one of which is called mevinolin, also known as lovastatin, which can successfully lower cholesterol and has created interest in both the natural and conventional health fields. While extracts of red yeast rice have been used in prescription drugs like Mevacor, natural supplements are now available and may afford the consumer a way to lower cholesterol without resorting to synthetic drug preparations. This is good news for people who suffer from moderately elevated cholesterol levels and are looking to natural remedies.

We are all aware by now that a high serum cholesterol level predisposes us to cardiovascular disease as well as other degenerative conditions. Learning to control our cholesterol levels, especially LDL and blood triglyceride levels, while keeping our HDL cholesterol at desirable levels can be rather frustrating. Naturally, we can decrease our consumption of animal fats and certain types of oils, eat more fiber and take prescription drugs to accomplish this objective. While dietary changes should be targeted first, turning to cholesterol-lowering prescription drugs has its pros and cons. These pharmaceutical preparations come with considerable side effects. Some of the most effective of these drugs contain enzymatic inhibitors which prevent cholesterol synthesis. Red yeast rice accomplishes the same enzyme inhibition but, unlike powerful drugs, is considered a natural alternative capable of safely promoting healthy serum cholesterol levels.

What Are Blood Lipids?

Cholesterol is an essential body lipid compound made by the liver. It can also be supplied from the diet by eating meat and dairy products. Cholesterol serves many life-giving functions and is necessary to our survival. Dietary cholesterol is only found in animal products and by-products. Excess cholesterol production raises blood cholesterol levels, which can ultimately lead to heart disease. Cholesterol is transported through the bloodstream via lipoproteins.

The fact that Eskimos eat a diet high in cholesterol from fish lipids and yet have a low incidence of cardiovascular disease suggests that perhaps we should concentrate more on the lipids we are lacking in our diet rather than on cholesterol consumption alone. Obviously, the relationship is a complex one. In other words, some people who eat diets high in cholesterol do not necessarily suffer from high blood cholesterol. On the other hand, others have a tendency to produce excess cholesterol in the liver if they eat animal-based foods.

It is important to understand that there are two types of cholesterol which affect our health in dramatically different ways. HDL (high density lipoprotein) is also called "good cholesterol" in that it transports cholesterol away from artery walls and back to the liver for storage. LDL (low density lipoprotein) is referred to as "bad cholesterol" because it promotes the circulation of cholesterol in the bloodstream, predisposing the arteries to plaque buildup and eventual blockage.

Triglycerides are fats that contain three groups of fatty acids: saturated, monounsaturated, and polyunsaturated. Saturated fats are considered the culprit fats and include butter, whole milk, sour cream, cheese and fats found in meats. (*Note:* Eating too much sugar can create excess insulin response, which may also raise blood lipids.) Hydrogenated fats have recently emerged as risky in that they contain trans-fatty acids which may also contribute to atherosclerosis. These are fats, which are normally liquid in form, have to undergo a process to make them solid which creates potentially dangerous by-products. Some margarines and shortenings fall into this category.

Monounsaturated and polyunsaturated fats do not raise blood cholesterol levels, Two recommended monounsaturated oils include canola and olive oil. Safflower and corn oil are highest in polyunsaturated fats. Current research suggests that cooking with monounsaturates is preferred.

While it is a well-established fact now that a low-fat diet can result in overall health improvement, people who restrict their fat intake to 10 or 12 percent often deprive themselves of essential fatty acids which are crucial to proper cellular metabolism and hormone synthesis. All fats are not bad. Eating the wrong kinds of fats can also promote a deficiency in essential fatty acids. It is crucial that we supplement our diets with these acids in the form of either fish oil, evening primrose, flaxseed oil, or GLA. A good blend of several of these oils is ideal.

WHAT RISKS DOES A HIGH CHOLESTEROL LEVEL POSE?

According to recent data, over 35 million Americans have a total serum cholesterol count over 240, which puts them at risk for cardiovascular disease. Interestingly, even if your cholesterol count falls in the range of 200-239, as it does for over 55 million people, your risk of heart disease is double that of individuals whose cholesterol levels are below 200. Naturally, genetic predisposition and the ratio of LDL cholesterol to HDL also determines who will develop coronary disease. High cholesterol, however, is considered a major predictor of cardiovascular disease. High cholesterol levels can also contribute to gallstones, impotence, mental impairment and hypertension.

Remember that you should always take more than one reading on two different occasions. If you are free of coronary artery disease, a desirable reading in total cholesterol is seen as less than 200 mg per 100 ml. Borderline readings range from 200 to 239. If you fall into this area, dietary changes and the use of certain supplements may be enough. Anything over 240 is considered high and may prompt your doctor to advise using cholesterol-lowering drugs. The ratio of LDL (bad cholesterol) to HDL (good cholesterol) is even more important than the total cholesterol reading. A high risk LDL count is over 160, borderline is from 130 to 159, and desirable levels are less than 130. If you have coronary artery disease, you should keep your LDL levels down to less than 100 mg/dL. Keep in mind that even if your total cholesterol count is acceptable and you lack in HDL, you may need some dietary adjustments. HDL readings less than 35 mg/dL are considered risky.

CHOLESTEROL LEVELS AND CORONARY HEART DISEASE

Coronary heart disease (CHD) refers to damage done to the heart when the coronary arteries become blocked or narrowed due to a buildup of plaque or oxidized cholesterol. Even more serious is the occasion when cholesterol buildup breaks off and lodges in the heart or the brain causing heart attack or stroke.

Coronary heart disease is an extremely common disorder of developed nations and causes more deaths in the United States than any other disease. Ironically, many people who die from heart disease are in otherwise good health. Like high blood pressure, which is a related disorder, heart disease can be a silent killer. Symptoms of CHD are impotence, heart attack or stroke. While mortality rates from CHD have declined over the last 20 years, data tells us that the reason for this decline is due to better medical technology. CHD claims more than one million deaths every year. The number of Americans with heart and artery disease is estimated around 50 million.

During the last two decades the public has been made aware of the importance of watching our cholesterol levels.

We have been given dietary guidelines to help us prevent heart disease. However, many of us have failed to become motivated to make the kind of dietary changes that could literally save our lives. The major causes of coronary heart disease include:

- obesity
- smoking
- high protein, high saturated fat diet
- lack of exercise
- high blood pressure
- high cholesterol levels
- genetic predisposition

PHARMACEUTICAL AGENTS vs. NATURAL COMPOUNDS

Using diet and natural supplements is the ideal method to reach and maintain healthy cholesterol levels. However, several drugs are available which lower cholesterol levels. These drugs include Cholestyramine, Gemfibrozil, Probucol, Mevacor, and even aspirin. These drugs all have side effects that should be considered. Liver problems, gastrointestinal ailments such as diarrhea, nausea and abdominal pain, muscle cramps, or skin rashes are a few of the known side effects of these drugs. Even in the case of prescription drugs which use compounds isolated from yeast sources, the medicinal compound is synthesized in a way which potentiates its action as well as its side effects. For this reason, using natural compounds like red yeast rice is considered less risky.

Unfortunately, as scientists examined plant chemistry, they had a tendency to isolate what they considered the most active compound and then artificially reproduce it.

Frequently, when the active principle of a phytomedicine is isolated, such as the mevinolin from red yeast rice, the synergistic, balancing effect of the entire phytochemical is lost.

Granted, the newly-created drug may be more potent and easier to ingest; however, the human body has a tendency to recognize it as a foreign and unnatural substance. As a result, a chain of physiological reactions occurs characterized by undesirable effects. Frequently, the body reacts to synthetic and powerful compounds much as it would to a poison.

By artificially refining or synthesizing various compounds in order to create a drug, toxicity can result. In other words, artificial compounds may offer valuable therapeutic benefits, but they usually cause a number of unwanted reactions as well. Unlike synthetic drugs, natural compounds work more in tandem with the body's natural processes, thereby avoiding many detrimental side effects associated with prescriptions. It is important to remember, however, that unlike the potent effects of synthetic drugs or analogs, natural compounds usually work more slowly. Of course, just because something is considered natural does not mean it can be used at will. Respecting natural medicines and using them properly is the key to success. Likewise, prescription drugs can be lifesavers but should only be used as a last resort.

Red Yeast Rice: A Definition

Red yeast rice refers to *Monascus purpureus,* or rice that has been fermented by the addition of yeast. Red yeast rice is incorporated into natural dietary supplements. It contains HMG-CoA (hydroxymethylglutaryl CoA) reductase inhibitors, which are compounds that inhibit an enzymatic reaction necessary to produce cholesterol in the body, especially in the liver. The liver is considered the main site of cholesterol production and is responsible for over 75 percent of our total cholesterol supply. The liver contains plenty of HMG-CoA reductase and red yeast rice works to inhibit its action, thereby decreasing cholesterol production. Several scientific studies have confirmed the ability of red yeast rice to reduce total cholesterol by very significant percentages. Red yeast rice also contains unsaturated fatty acids that may also help reduce serum lipids or blood fats we call triglycerides.

USAGE

Red yeast rice supplements are designed for those individuals who suffer from moderately high cholesterol levels. Supplements should be incorporated into an overall therapeutic strategy utilizing diet and exercise. Red yeast rice supplements should not be viewed as a cure for any condition, but rather as a natural way to help maintain desirable cholesterol levels. Anyone with high cholesterol levels should see their physician. If your cholesterol level is above 230, talk to your doctor about trying red yeast rice therapy before going on prescription drugs.

A BRIEF HISTORICAL PERSPECTIVE

Red yeast rice enjoys a long history of use in Asian cuisine for centuries dating back to 800 A.D. In south China, red yeast rice has been consumed as both a food stuff and medicinal agent for over two millennia. Records dating back to the fourteenth century describe its use for the treatment of several maladies including infections, circulatory problems and stomach ailments. More recently, cultures in Japan, Thailand,

India, Korea and even the Philippines use red yeast rice in both cookery and as a therapeutic compound. Over the last few decades its popularity has taken hold in European countries such as Germany.

Today, red yeast is routinely used to give foods a rich, stable red color. Meat products, poultry, fish, ketchup, chocolates, cereals, jams, and beverages have been colored with red yeast pigments. The advantages of using red yeast to give foods color is that it is considered nontoxic and remains stable even when exposed to high temperatures.

As far as its medicinal value, scientists have isolated and classified various species of the proprietary strain *Monascus* from red yeast. Scientific research confirms the pharmacologic qualities of this substance, especially in regard to the reduction of LDL cholesterol (bad cholesterol) and blood triglycerides or fats. Asians eat between 14 and 55 grams of red yeast daily sprinkling it on other main dishes like tofu as a colorful topping.

Red Yeast Rice and Prescription Drugs for Cholesterol

In 1980, a Japanese scientist isolated a metabolite of red yeast that significantly reduced artificially-induced high cholesterol levels in laboratory test rats. One of these extracts, monacolin (from the word *monascus*), is regarded as a cholesterol-reducing medicine. When monacolin was discovered, it was not registered. Later this same compound became the basis for a number of drugs under various trade names worldwide, including lovastatin, simvastatin, pravasin, and mevastatin. Presently, extracts or capsulized *Monascus* is sold in Japan as monacolin and is considered a dietary supplement that, according to a Japanese patent, also helps to lower high blood pressure.

LOVASTATIN AND MEVINOLIN

Apparently, in previous tests designed to isolate metabolites from fungal strains, compounds were discovered found which had the ability to lower cholesterol. Unfortunately, these substances were also considered highly toxic; therefore their ability to decrease cholesterol was not applicable. The notion, however, that another metabolite could be found that had the ability to treat high cholesterol by blocking the action of HMG-CoA reductase without any toxicity motivated additional research.

Subsequently, scientists were able to isolate lovastatin from a fungal strain of *Aspergillus terrus* and later introduced the first HMG-CoA reductase inhibitor into the pharmaceutical market. Even though this compound, known as monacolin, had actually been isolated years before from *Monascus*, its structure was never formally registered. As a result, scientists had the option to file for a patent and begin marketing this compound now called lovastatin for coronary heart disease.

Lovastatin is the generic name of the prescription drug called Mevacor. The success of lovastatin prompted the quest to find other compounds extracted from fungal strains that could inhibit HMG-CoA reductase. Moreover, other chemical compounds were derived from lovastatin in an attempt to synthesize a superior product. Simvastatin, another cholesterol-lowering drug, is a methyl derivative of lovastatin. Pravastatin was also categorized as an HMG-CoA reductase inhibitor. Lovastatin's therapeutic action is due to the fact that it converts to mevinolin in the body. Mevinolin is the active principle found in red yeast rice.

Mevinolin not only lowers cholesterol but has some antioxidant properties as well. Mevinolin enzymatically inhibits a compound called mevalonate, which ends up decreasing LDL cholesterol (the bad kind) while either maintaining or increasing HDL cholesterol (the good kind). The chemical structure of mevinolinic acid is similar to HMG-CoA. As a result, mevinolinic acid competes with HMG-CoA for HMG-CoA reductase. Consequently, the enzyme activity that produces mevalonic acid, a precursor of cholesterol, is decreased.

The Scientific Validation of Red Yeast Rice

The bulk of research supporting the use of red yeast rice for cholesterol levels has been conducted by Chinese scientists, although American studies are thought to be underway at this writing. While medical practitioners are typically reticent about accepting data from foreign sources, some of the 20 studies published did use placebo-controls and double-blind formats. All of these trials involved a great number of individuals and found that red yeast rice can lower cholesterol counts from 20 to 40 points when combined with diet and exercise. The first American study on red yeast rice using Cholestin, a commercial dietary supplement, was conducted at UCLA and supports the idea that red yeast rice can accomplish far more than just dietary or exercise changes. People with moderately high cholesterol who took the dietary supplement lowered cholesterol levels by an average of 40 points, as reported by a study presented at the Experimental Biology Conference in San Francisco (Hellmich). Both animal and human studies support the ability of red yeast rice to effectively lower serum lipid levels.

THE WANG STUDY

J. Wang and his staff performed a randomized, single-blind trial in 502 patients who were diagnosed with high cholesterol and triglyceride levels. These test subjects had a serum total cholesterol greater than or equal to 230, an LDL count greater than or equal to 130, or triglycerides values ranging from 200-400. These participants also had an HDL count less than or equal to 40 for men and 45 for women. Patients were then randomly divided into one of four groups: groups A, C, and D were the treatment groups and group B was the control group. Patients in the treatment groups were given 600 mg of red yeast rice twice a day (1200 mg/d) whereas the patients in the control group were given a Chinese herb called Jiaogulan which had reputed cholesterol-lowering properties. After four weeks of therapy with red yeast rice, total cholesterol levels decreased by 17.1 percent whereas the reduction of total cholesterol in the control group was 4.8 percent. Moreover, LDL count in the red yeast rice group was reduced by an average of 24.6 percent versus an average of 6.3 percent in the control group. Serum triglycerides decreased by an average of 19.8 percent in the treatment group and 9.2 percent in the control group. In addition, HDL levels increased by 12.8 percent with red yeast rice and 4.9 percent without.

At the end of eight weeks of treatment, the patients in the treatment group had an impressive average reduction in total cholesterol of 22.7 percent versus an average reduction of 7 percent in the control group. Red yeast rice supplementation had reduced their LDL levels by 30.9 percent. This reduction was significantly greater than that in the control group. Total blood triglyceride reduction was reduced by 34.1 percent with the red yeast rice and 12.8 percent without. Of additional interest is the fact that any adverse reaction to the red yeast rice was rare and considered mild and was quickly resolved.

Those that orchestrated this study came to the conclusion that red yeast rice is a "highly effective and well tolerated dietary supplement that can be used to regulate elevated serum cholesterol and triglycerides" (Wang).

RED YEAST RICE AND TUMORS

One of the clinical studies conducted at the College of Pharmacy of Nihon University in Japan found that red yeast rice pigment, referred to as *Monascus* pigment, was able to inhibit the growth of malignant tumors induced in laboratory test mice. These scientists extracted the monascus pigment from red malted rice and administered it orally. What they concluded was that this red pigment did indeed have the ability to suppress skin tumors in test mice (Yasukawa).

THE PRESERVING PROPERTIES
OF RED YEAST

The preserving effect of *Monascus* ferment from red yeast has been scientifically confirmed. *Monascus* is especially effective for conserving foodstuffs especially when it is combined with organic acids. Japanese patents describe the contents of *Monascus* and these acid compounds as a very effective preservative. Both components are mixed and added to food or fodder. This preserving effect has particular benefit in regards to the control of *Bacillus subtilis, Staphylococcus aureus* and other microbes. Experts are encouraging more research into using red yeast as an antibacterial agent to protect meat products. *Monascus* also possesses antifungal activity. For these reasons, some are advocating the use of red yeast in lieu of nitrates, which are commonly used to preserve foods like bacon, lunch meats, etc. Nitrites are considered potential carcinogens.

Safety Issues

While adverse effects have been rare and considered very mild, they have included heartburn, flatulence, and dizziness. If you choose to use a red yeast supplement, check your cholesterol levels after a two-month course of therapy. Anyone taking prescription drugs to control cholesterol levels should not take red yeast rice without their doctor's approval. In addition, people who suffer from yeast allergies or are experiencing liver disease or infection should not use red yeast supplements. Avoid red yeast rice supplements if you are pregnant or breast-feeding. If you have any preexisting condition or take drugs of any kind, check with your doctor or health care practitioner before taking red yeast rice to avoid any adverse interactions. If you are currently taking cholesterol-lowering prescription drugs, don't stop taking them or alter their dosage in any way without consulting your physician. Children should not take this supplement unless advised to do so by their physician.

Recently there has been some speculation that the *Monascus* fungus may also contain a fungal toxin called citrinin, which is related to penicillium. This concern is considered weak and unfounded by many experts who point out that red yeast rice has been used for decades and poses no health threat.

A long-term Japanese study concluded that *Monascus* could be safely used. It has been used extensively in Germany and other European countries for its ability to color foods and is considered perfectly safe. Because red yeast rice has such a long history of use and has also been the subject of intensive research, it is assumed that it can be taken safely in supplement or food additive form.

Red Yeast Rice Supplements: What's Out There

Red yeast rice supplements are now available on the U.S. market. Look for products that are in a concentrate form and contain a standardized minimum percentage of mevinolin. Powdered extracts are available. Making sure your supplement has guaranteed potency and comes from a reliable distributor is essential. Finding a reasonably priced product that is convenient to take is also recommended. Red yeast rice supplements may also be found under the label "hongqu."

Red Yeast Rice, Legal Issues and the FDA

Last November, the FDA (Food and Drug Administration) decided that Cholestin, which is the product name of a supplement containing red yeast rice, should be considered an unapproved new drug. The FDA based its case on the fact that red yeast rice contains mevinolin, a substance the agency saw as identical to lovastatin, which is the active component of the prescription drug called Mevacor.

A ban of Cholestin and red yeast rice was set into motion and importation of red yeast rice was blocked. As a result of the ban, a preliminary injunction against the FDA was brought forth by the company which manufactured Cholestin. Fortunately, after serious questions were raised regarding the legality of the FDA's stance and interpretation of the Dietary Supplement Health and Education Act (DSHEA), a federal judge in Utah recently issued a preliminary injunction on the ban of the supplement Cholestin.

Michael Q. Ford, executive director of the National Nutritional Foods Association, was delighted by this action. It was seen as a victory for both suppliers and consumers of natural, dietary supplements. Subsequently, a U.S. District Court Judge stressed that the FDA did not consider Cholestin or red yeast rice to pose any potential health risks. Once again the legal definition of "dietary supplement" comes into play in this scenario. The reference of red yeast rice or Cholestin as an "article" created confusion and ultimately led to the conclusion that the FDA was using the term "article" to indict natural compounds that may also be found in prescription drugs, thereby banning their sale or importation. The legality of their definition of red yeast rice was seriously questioned.

As it stands now, red yeast rice can be imported for use in dietary supplements, a freedom which is considered a victory for health-conscious individuals everywhere. The fact that red yeast rice, or hongqu, is listed in the *Materia Medica* also supports its definition as an herbal medicine and technically designates it as a dietary supplement not subject to FDA regulation.

Dietary Guidelines for Cholesterol Management

Our consumption of dietary cholesterol has been considered one of the most significant factors in determining whether we will develop heart disease. As a result, many of us replaced butter with polyunsaturated margarine, stopped eating eggs, and gave up a variety of meat products when we were told that animal fats were not desirable. Now, as is frequently the case, new data is telling us that high levels of cholesterol are not solely the result of eating foods like butter and eggs, but are due to a variety of factors. Eating whole foods as nature designed them should not hurt our bodies. The enormous consumption of processed fats, refined foods and the lack of fiber, however, has upset our biological safeguards resulting in disrupted physiological balances.

Perhaps it's not so important to totally eliminate certain foods as it is to balance them or use them in moderation. Ancel Keys observed that the much higher content of plasma cholesterol levels of men in Minnesota as compared to Naples, Italy could not be explained by patterns of fatty acid or cholesterol intake. His study indicated that the Italians ate diets high in cereals, vegetables, legumes and fruits which seemed to control cholesterol levels even if they ate butter, meat, etc. (Schweizer). Naturally, if we suffer from elevated cholesterol, we need to limit our consumption of animal fats. It is also true, however, that using the right supplements and foods together helps to balance and control cholesterol in the way that Mother Nature intended.

SPECIFIC SUGGESTIONS

Keep these facts in mind when designing a dietary approach to cholesterol control. Generally speaking, it is always good to emphasize a lower fat, higher fiber diet. Eat plenty of oat bran, fruits and vegetables such as bananas, apples, melons, broccoli, cabbage, green leafy vegetables, peas, prunes, beets, carrots, and spinach. Avoid or limit the following foods: smoked or aged cheeses and meats, chocolate, animal fats, gravies, broths, and processed foods. Watch your intake of white sugar and caffeine. Use olive and flaxseed oil and limit saturated (animal) and hydrogenated fats (margarines). Eat soy foods such as tofu. Coldwater fish and lean white meats are also recommended. Use olive and canola oil and stay away from hydrogenated fats. Exercise is also an integral component to maintaining good cardiovascular health and should be implemented under the guidelines set by your physician.

THE FIBER COMPONENT

Foods that are rich in fiber such as oats and beans, gums, pectins and psyllium all significantly lower blood fats or cholesterol levels. When you eat a lot of fiber, you get rid of more bile. When less bile is returned to the liver, it kicks in and makes more bile acids which uses up cholesterol floating around in your blood, which lowers your cholesterol level (Story). Fiber also influences the secretion if insulin which has a bearing on how lipids are broken down in the bloodstream and stored (Kritchevsky).

Nearly a dozen studies conducted over the past decade have proven that oat bran lowers cholesterol levels. Soluble-fiber cereals are highly recommended as bad cholesterol busters. In addition, psyllium has also proven itself to be a cholesterol inhibitor (Lipsky). The *Journal of the American Medical Association* stated in 1988, "A broad public health approach to lowered cholesterol levels by additional dietary modifications, such as with soluble fiber, may be preferred to a medically oriented campaign that focuses on drug therapy" (Kinosian).

At this writing, we have accrued plenty of data that dietary fiber can lower blood lipids and decrease our risk of heart attack or stroke. Combining fiber with supplementation and dietary changes provides an excellent strategy for good cardiovascular health.

Note: Do not take any fiber supplement at the same time you take your other nutrient supplements to avoid any interference with fat-soluble vitamins, etc.

RED YEAST RICE: COMPLEMENTARY NUTRIENTS

The following list of nutrients can work in conjunction with red yeast rice supplements to control cholesterol levels. Please remember to consult your physician prior to taking any of these supplements:

GARLIC (ALLIUM SATIVUM): Pure powdered extracts are recommended and can help lower high cholesterol or blood lipids (Lau).

COENZYME Q10: Helps to strengthen and oxygenate heart muscle and contributes to metabolic processes (Yamagami).

NIACIN: May help to increase HDL cholesterol (good cholesterol) and improve the total cholesterol/HDL ratio (DiPalma).

ESSENTIAL FATTY ACIDS (OMEGA-3 AND OMEGA-6): Both of these fatty acids which are found in fish oils and oils like flaxseed, can contribute to decreased blood pressure and blood lipids. The fact that Eskimo cultures eat diets high in saturated fats but have low cardiovascular disease is attributed to the effect of coldwater fish consumption (Singer).

VITAMIN E: Works to scavenge for free radicals and helps to protect against heart disease and stroke by also reducing LDL cholesterol. Low levels of this vitamin are considered a primary predictor of heart disease (Gey).

FIBER SUPPLEMENT: Boosting soluble fiber intake can be one of the most effective treatments for high blood cholesterol levels when combined with dietary changes and other natural compounds (Little).

CHITOSAN: A form of fiber that absorbs dietary fat in the gut and can also inhibit LDL cholesterol (bad cholesterol) while boosting desirable HDL cholesterol levels (Vahouny).

LECITHIN: This compound contains choline which works to increase bile solubility and lower cholesterol levels.

CHROMIUM: Studies have conclusively shown that chromium supplementation does indeed lower elevated blood cholesterol and triglyceride levels.

GINGER: Studies have found that ginger can reduce cholesterol levels by inhibiting its absorption.

SOY ISOFLAVONES AND SOY PROTEIN: These compounds (especially one called genistein) can help to control cholesterol levels.

STRESS AND HIGH CHOLESTEROL

Scientific research suggests that stress may raise blood cholesterol. Some people seem to oxidize cholesterol differently when under stress due to the release of chemicals like epinephrine and cortisol. These stress hormones can cause abnormal oxidative processes which enable cholesterol or plaque to more readily adhere to artery walls. In addition, these hormones can cause the release of an amino acid which also impairs cholesterol metabolism. There is little question that unmanaged stress contributes to plaque formation and obstruction. Learning to deal with stress is so important in controlling both high blood pressure and high cholesterol. Exercise, controlled breathing, meditation and disciplines like yoga can be of tremendous value in helping to lower stress levels.

ADDITIONAL SUGGESTIONS

• Stop smoking. A definite link exists between smoking and coronary artery disease which can also cause high blood pressure.
• Learn to relax and fight stress. Use breathing techniques, yoga, exercise, music, etc. to inhibit tension. When you feel tense, stop and use visualization techniques to achieve tranquillity. Slow down if your pace of living has become too stressful.
• Use olive, canola and flaxseed oils and take an essential fatty acid supplement daily.
• Eat plenty of fish.
• Keep your diet low in hydrogenated and saturated fat and salt and high in fiber and fresh fruits and vegetables.
• Keep your weight down and exercise regularly.

• Do not consume alcohol.
• Do not consume caffeine, especially in the form of coffee.

Afterword

A symposium on *Monascus* (red yeast) and its various applications will be held in Toulouse, France. The theme of the symposium is *Monascus* microbiology, biochemistry, genetics and biotechnology in general and will consist of keynote presentations by internationally acknowledged scientists. The symposium will be held in the Center for Unesco in Toulouse, France. Obviously, this natural compound is getting the attention of scientists everywhere. Red yeast rice is a natural compound which should be considered by anyone who has moderately elevated cholesterol levels. It has proven its ability to lower cholesterol and can do so without the potentially harmful side effects of prescription drugs. Combining red yeast therapy with dietary and lifestyle changes can certainly contribute to better cardiovascular health.

References

DiPalma, J.R. and W.S. Thayer, "The use of niacin as a drug," Ann Rev Nutr, 1991, 11: 169-87.

Fabre, C., A. Santerre and M. Loret, "Production and food application of the red pigments of Monascus Ruber," Journal of Food Science, Sept. 1993, 58: 1099.

Fong, W.F., S.H. Lai, Y.L. Wong-Leung and S.W. Chiu, "Food Processing Wastes as Fermentation Substrates for the Production of Monascus Yellow and Red Pigments," Proceedings of Symposium on Microbial and Engineering Techniques in Waste Treatment, Hong Kong, 122-132, Commercial Publishers, Hong Kong (1991).

Gey, K.F., et al., "Inverse correlation between plasma vitamin E and mortality from ischemic heart disease in cross-cultural epidemiology," Amer Jour Clin Nutri, 1991, 53: 326S- 334S.

Hellmich, Nanci, "Red yeast rice cuts 'bad' cholesterol in study at UCLA,"UMI Article Re. No.USA-2363-53.

Hossain, C.F., E. Okuyama and M. Yamazaki, "A new series of coumarin derivatives having monoamine oxidase inhibitory activity from Monascus anka," Faculty of Pharmaceutical Sciences, Chiba University, Japan. Chem Pharm Bull (Tokyo) Aug 1996, 44(8):1535-9.

Izawa, Satoko, Nanaho Harad and Toshirou Watanabe, "Inhibitory effects of food coloring agents derived from Monascus on the mutagenicity of hyerocylcic amines," Journal of Agri and Food Chem, Oct. 1997, 45: 3980-84.

Johnson, Ian, "Brewhaha: Fight Over Rice Yeast Pits Chinese Medicine Against Western Ways U.S. Firm Says Remedy Cuts Cholesterol, So the FDA Calls It a Drug in Disguise: Why Vague Labeling Helps," UMI Publication No.04816093, UMI Article Re. WSJ-2260-224.

Juzlova, P., T. Ruzanka and L. Martinkova, "Long chain fatty acids from Monascus purpureus," Phytochemistry, 1996, 43(1): 151-53.

Kinosian, B.P., and J.M. Eisenber, "Cutting into cholesterol. Cost-effective alternatives for treating hypercholesterolemia," Journal of the

American Medical Association, April 15, 1988: 259(15): 2249-54.

Kritchevsky, David and Charles Bonfield, Dietary Fiber in Health and Disease, St. Paul, Minnesota: Eagan Press, 1995.

Kromhout, D., "Dietary fiber and 10-year mortality for coronary heart disease, cancer and all causes," Lancet 1982: 2: 518-22.

Kuramoto Y; Yamada K; Tsuruta O; Sugano M, "Effect of natural food colorings on immunoglobulin production in vitro by rat spleen lymphocytes," Department of Food Science and Technology, Faculty of Agriculture, Kyushu University, Fukuoka, Japan.Biosci Biotechnol Biochem, Oct 1996, 60(10):1712-3.

Lau, B.H., et al., "Allium sativum (garlic) and atherosclerosis; A review," Nutri Res, 1983, (3): 119-128.

Li, Chang, Yan Zhu and Wang Yinye, "Monascus purpureus: fermented rice (red yeast rice): a natural food product that lowers blood cholesterol in animal models of hypercholesterolemia," Nutrition Research , Jan. 1998, 18: 71-81.

Little, P., et al., "A controlled trial of a low sodium, low fat, high fiber diet in treated hypertensive patients: the efficacy of multiple dietary intervention," Postgraduate Medical Journal, 1990, 66(778): 616-21.

Lipid-Lowering Effects of red yeast rice, No. 244 of Medical Sciences Bulletin, January 1998.

Lipsky, H., M. Gloger and W.H. Frishman, "Dietary Fiber for reducing blood cholesterol, Journal of Clinical Pharmacology, Aug. 1990, 30(8): 699-703.

Louria, D., et al., "Onion extract in treatment of hypertension and hyperlipidemia: A preliminary communication," Curr Ther Res, 1985, 37(1):127-31.

Martinkova, L., P. Juzlova and D. Vesely, "Biological activity of polyketide pigments produced by the fungus Monascus," Journal of Applied Bacteriology, Dec. 1995, 79: 609-16.

Schweizer, T.F., and C.A. Edwards, eds., Dietary Fibre, A Component of Food, Nutritional Function in Health and Disease, 322, London: Springer-Verlag, 1992.

Shinnick, F.L., et al., "Dose response to a dietary oat bran fraction in cholesterol-fed rats," Jour Nutri. 1990, 120(6): 561-68.

Singer, P., "Blood pressure-lowering effect of w-3 polyunsaturated fatty acids in clinical studies," in A.P. Simopoulos et al., eds. "Health effects of w-3 polyunsaturated fatty acids in seafoods," World Rev Nutr Diet, 1991, 66:329-48.

Stolberg, Sheryl Gay, "Drug Regulators Make Push To Rein In Herbal Remedies," New York Times Late Edition: (East Coast), Jun 10, 1998, UMI Publication No. 05082549.

Story, J.A., "Dietary Fiber and lipid metabolism," Medical Aspects of Dietary Fiber, 138, New York: Plenum Medical, 1980.

Uchida, S. et al., "Inhibitory effects of condensed tannins on angiotensin converting enzyme," Jap Jour Pharmacol, 1987, 43:242-5.

Vahouny, George, et al., "Comparative effects of chitosan and cholestryramine on lymphatic absorption of lipids in the rat," Amer Jour Clinical Nutri, 1983, 38(2): 278-84.

Wang J, Zongliang L, Chi J, et al., "Multi center clinical trial of the serum lipid-lowering effects of a Monascus Purpureus (red yeast) rice preparation from traditional Chinese medicine," Current Therapeutic Research ,1997, 58(12):964-78.

Wong, W.F., Fong and W.L. Lam, "Production of -Galactosidase by Monascus Grown on Soybean and Sugar Cane Wastes", World Journal of Microbiology and Biotechnology, 1993, (5)529-533.

Yamagami, T., et al., "Bioenergetics in clinical medicine: Studies on coenzyme Q-10 and essential hypertension," Res Commun Chem Pathol Pharmacol, 1975, 11:273.

Yasukawa, K., M. Takahashi and S. Yamanouchi , "Inhibitory effect of oral administration of Monascus pigment on tumor promotion in two-stage carcinogenesis in mouse skin" College of Pharmacy, Nihon University, Chiba, Japan. Oncology 1996 May-Jun, 53(3):247-9.